ISBN: 978-09967704-6-0

Library of Congress Control Number: 2020946287

Author: Rimona Seay
Illustrator: Rimona Seay
Editor: Brett Lark
Book Design: Russell G. Baker

Printed and bound in the United States of America
First printed October 2020

Published by Brett Lark, LLC
333 N 7th St #A
Burbank, CA 91501

The Vegan Crocodile

By Rimona Seay

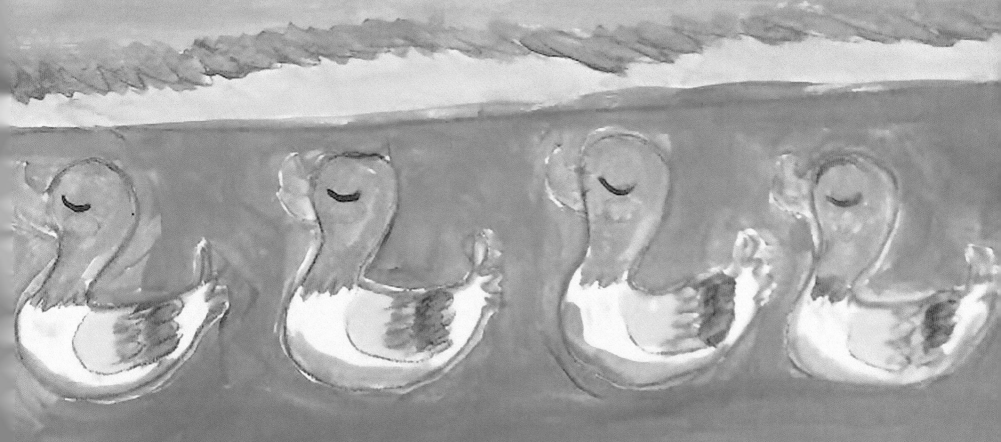

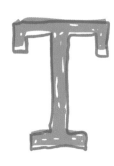oday, the Duck family is very happy, indeed. It is a big day because the last born duck is ready for his first swim. Mama Duck is very worried for him and repeats the rules to him and the rest of her ducklings:

"Listen to me all of you. Especially you, my Baby Duck. Stay well within the group. Do not stray or else you might be lost.

There is danger in the water—strange creatures and crocodiles with ferocious teeth that would eat you up in one swallow. If you get tired, tell me and we shall all stop to wait for you."

"Yes, mamma. We will be very careful. We will follow you without getting lost," the little ducklings wagged.

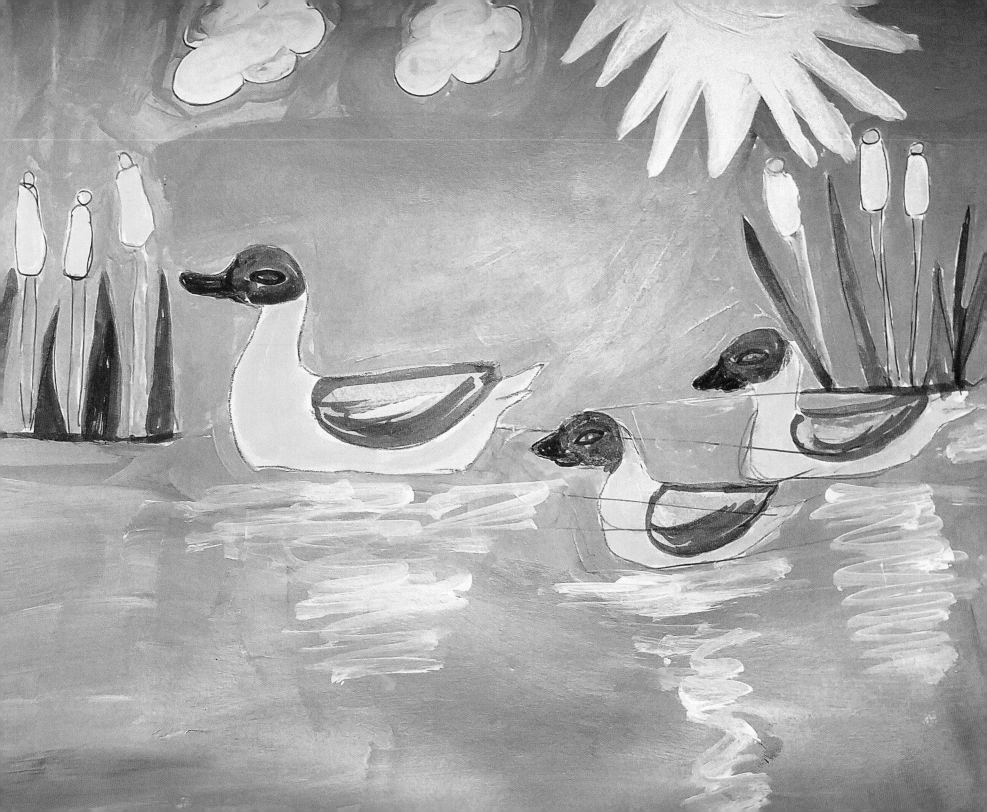

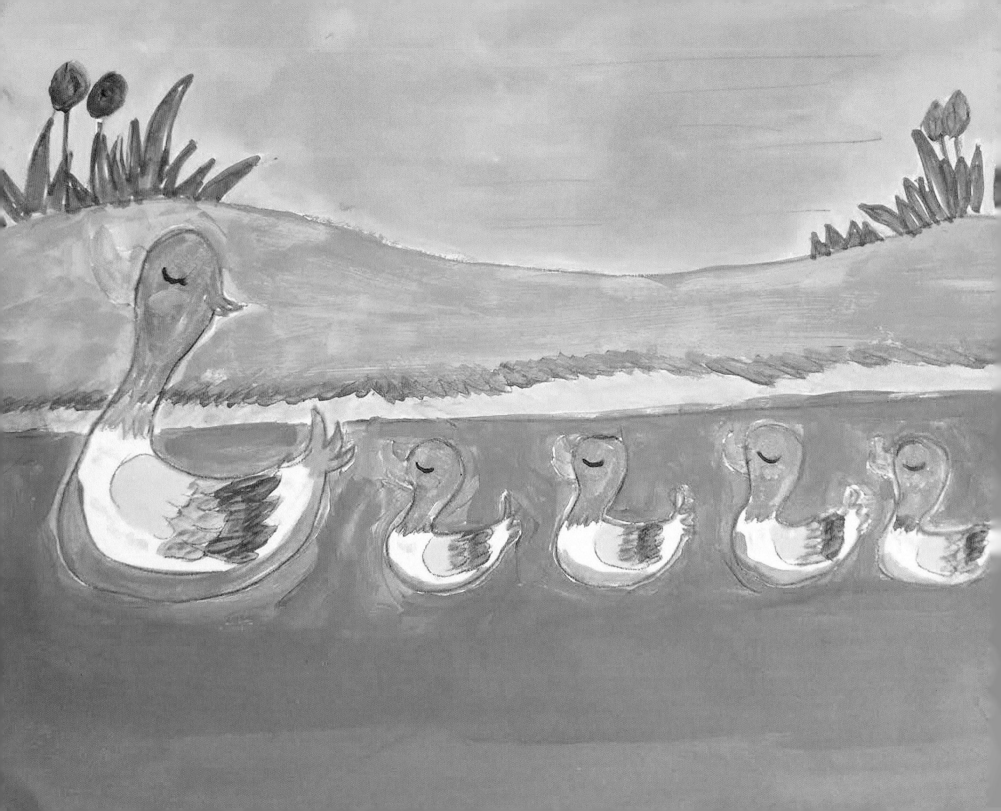

"Okay then. Come on children. Put yourself one behind the other and follow me. It's a beautiful day today, a great day to have some fun," quacked Mama Duck.

All the ducklings lined up behind Mama Duck and all began swimming. It was a beautiful day! Each duckling seemed to keep Mama Duck's pace. Baby Duck was dazzled by all the new sights.

Soon, Baby Duck began feeling a bit tired. He thought about telling Mama that he felt winded and needed a break, but he was too proud to say anything. So instead, he decided to slow down a little to rest his duck legs and enjoy the scenery. The water was soft. The sky was blue. Tree branches touched the surface of the water softly, making small waves, and the birds flew so low that he wondered if he could catch one.

Baby Duck became so involved in his contemplations that soon he looked for his family and realized that he was very, very, lost. Baby Duck was all alone in the water and his family was no where to be seen. Baby Duck began to panic and started swimming very quickly. He hoped that if he swam at a quick rate, he would be able to catch up with his family in no time.

After a while, he realized that there was nobody around him. He began to worry. "What's going to happen to me?" cried Baby Duck.

Suddenly, he felt the water moving around him. Two very large yellow eyes surfaced and looked right at Baby Duck. Panicked, he tried to flap his little wings, but he hadn't learned how to fly yet.

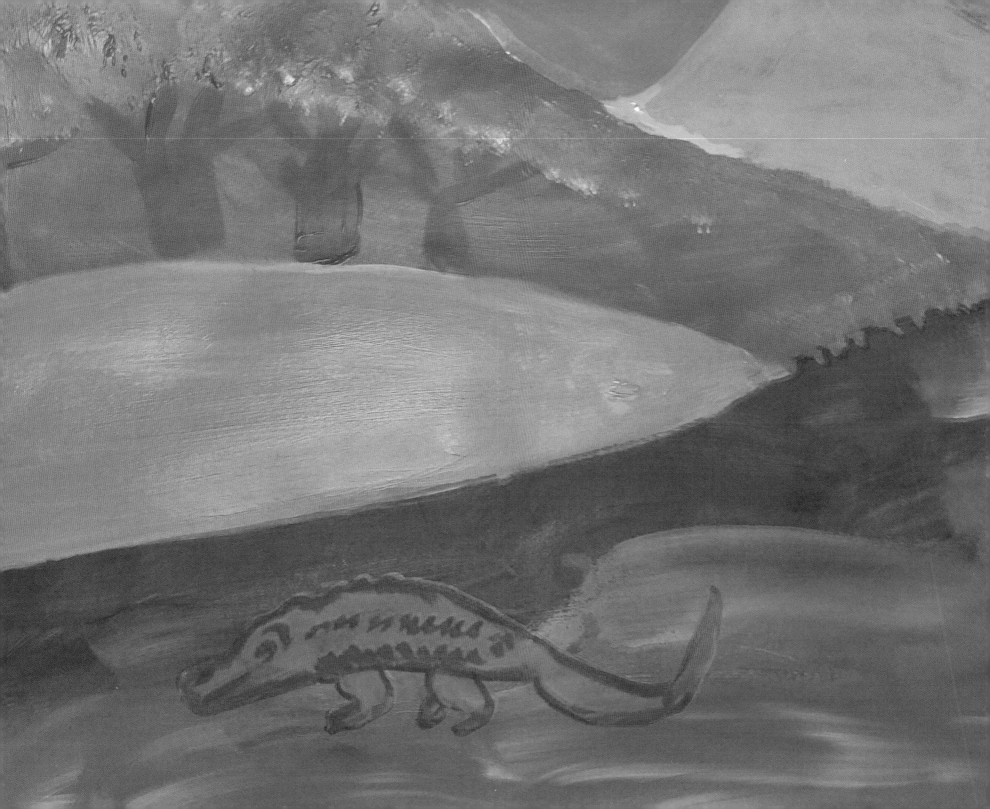

Soon Baby Duck found himself perched on the back of a big green animal rising out of the water. Baby Duck wondered if this was one of the dangerous creatures his mother had told him about. He tried not to think of what might happen to him.

The large crocodile looked at him and gently asked, "What are you doing out here all alone? Where's your family?" The Baby Duck nervously replied, "I d-d-do not know."

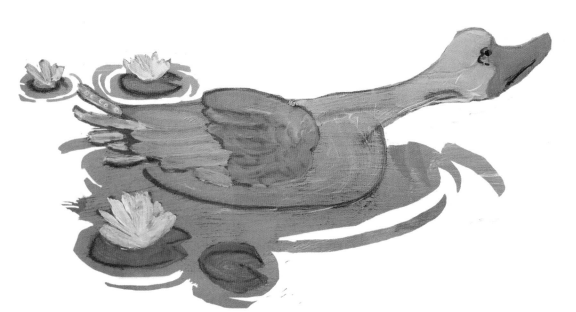

"I'm lost," Baby Duck said sadly. "Who are you?"

"I am Mr. Crocodile," Mr. Crocodile said with kindness in his voice.

'Oh no!' thought Baby Duck. His mother had told him that crocodiles were dangerous with ferocious teeth that would eat baby ducks in one swallow.

"Are you going to eat me?" Baby Duck asked.

"No, my little one." replied the crocodile with a soft laugh.
"Do not worry. I'm a vegan crocodile."

"Vegan? What is that?" Baby Duck asked, still not feeling safe on the back of a large green crocodile.

"Well, it means I eat herbs, but no meat—not animals, like Ducks. So do not worry. We are both going to find your family. I can swim pretty fast, so hang on!"

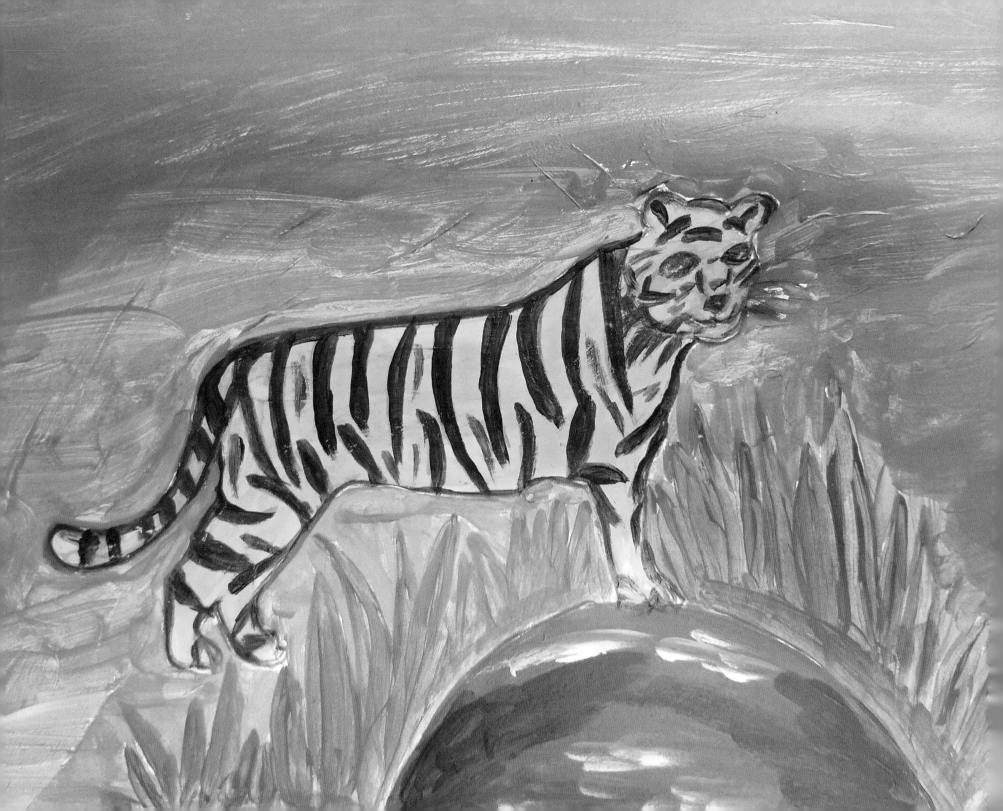

At the edge of the water, a tiger had spotted the baby duck. He licked his lips at the idea of swallowing the little duck whole. The tiger was very sly and came up with a plan.

He approached the shore and asked the crocodile, "Well, dear friend, what are you doing with a duck on your back? Why don't you swallow it?"

The crocodile did not like the tiger's tone and knew very well that it was dangerous to approach him. Nevertheless, he opened wide his mouth to show his big, sharp fangs and replied, "He lost his mother and my mission is to get him reunited with his family. If you come too close, I'll bite you on the nose with my teeth!"

The tiger drew back quickly and snarly replied. "Oh, but of course, I will leave you two," thinking to himself that if he followed the crocodile discreetly, he could find the entire duck family and have a duck feast.

The crocodile continued his search for the duck family. While swimming, a long neck giraffe drinking at the edge of the water took a glimpse at the curious scene.

"Hello, my friend! Well, you have a new companion I see? But what is he doing there, on your back? Why do you not eat that little duck?" inquired Madam Giraffe.

"Ah, well, I am after all a vegan crocodile, Madam Giraffe, and this little duck has lost his mother. I have a mission to find his family!" explained the vegan crocodile.

"Then I'll help you. I am tall and my long neck will allow me to see far beyond the tree-tops to help spot his family!" offered Madam Giraffe.

And so, baby duck on the back of the vegan crocodile, led by Madam Giraffe (and secretly followed by the sly tiger, of course), set off on their journey.

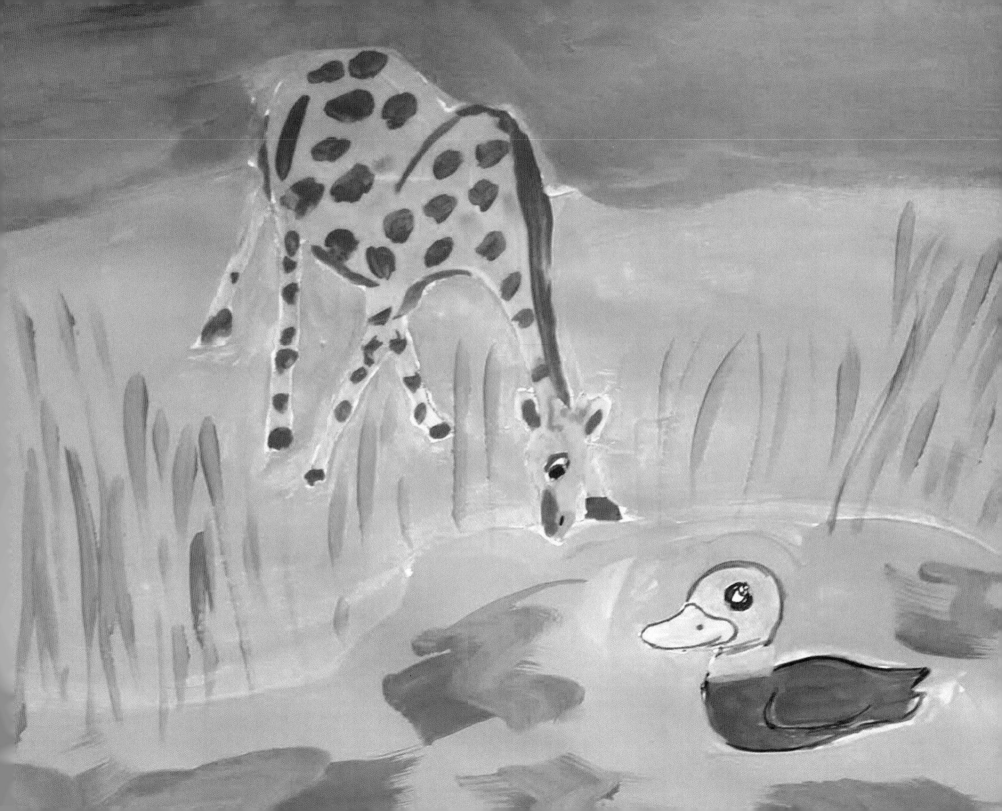

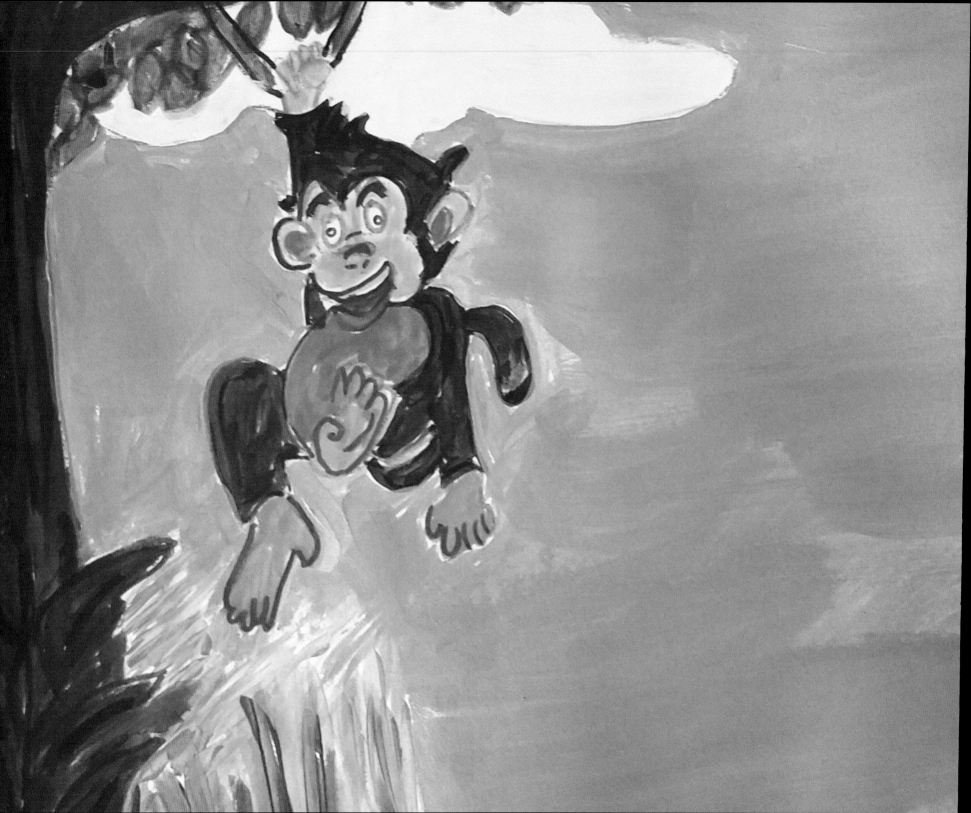

The giraffe continued scanning high above the trees but no duck family could be seen. While searching a curious monkey perched on a tree had observed the odd looking trio with a duck riding on a crocodile's back. Wishing to know more he swung over to the group and asked the crocodile.

"I say sir, are you aware there is a duckling on your back? Why do you not eat him with your sharp teeth?" asked Sir Monkey.

"Well, a baby duckling wouldn't do as food for a vegan crocodile. These teeth only bite plants and sweet tasting fruits. Besides, we are helping this baby duck find his family!" informed the vegan crocodile.

"In that case, I can help," replied the monkey. "I can climb in the trees and jump from branch to branch to inform the family when Madam Giraffe has found them."

As the four continued on their mission, Madam Giraffe scanned the waters high above the trees and her neck was getting tired. Suddenly, she spotted the Duck family! "I see your family little duck! They are down the river a ways further!" cried Madam Giraffe.

"Wonderful!" rejoiced the vegan crocodile. "Sir Monkey, please swing up ahead to let the Duck family know that we are on our way and to wait for us."

"It would be my pleasure," assured Sir Monkey. And with that Sir Monkey swung out of sight to tell the Duck family about their missing baby.

"Yay!" Baby Duck exclaimed. "Thank you, Madam Giraffe, for looking for my family."

Madam Giraffe blushed and kicked some sand next to her. "Awe, you are quite welcome." And the intrepid trio continued down the river toward the Duck Family as Sir Monkey swung from tree to tree in-front of them and out of sight.

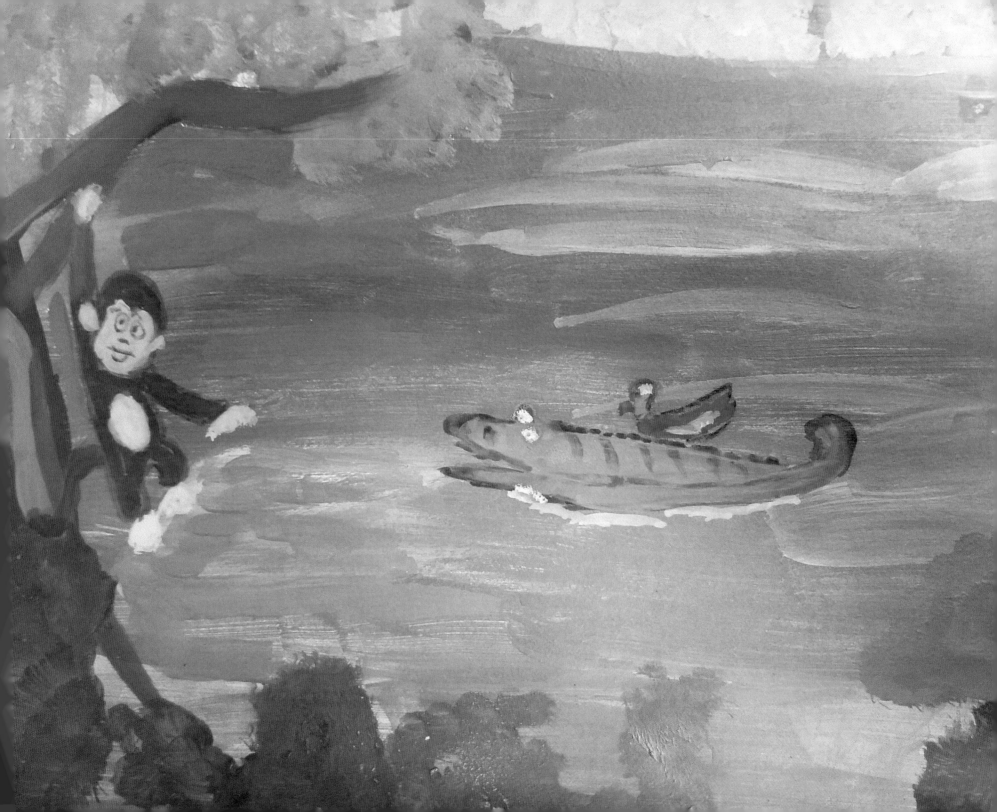

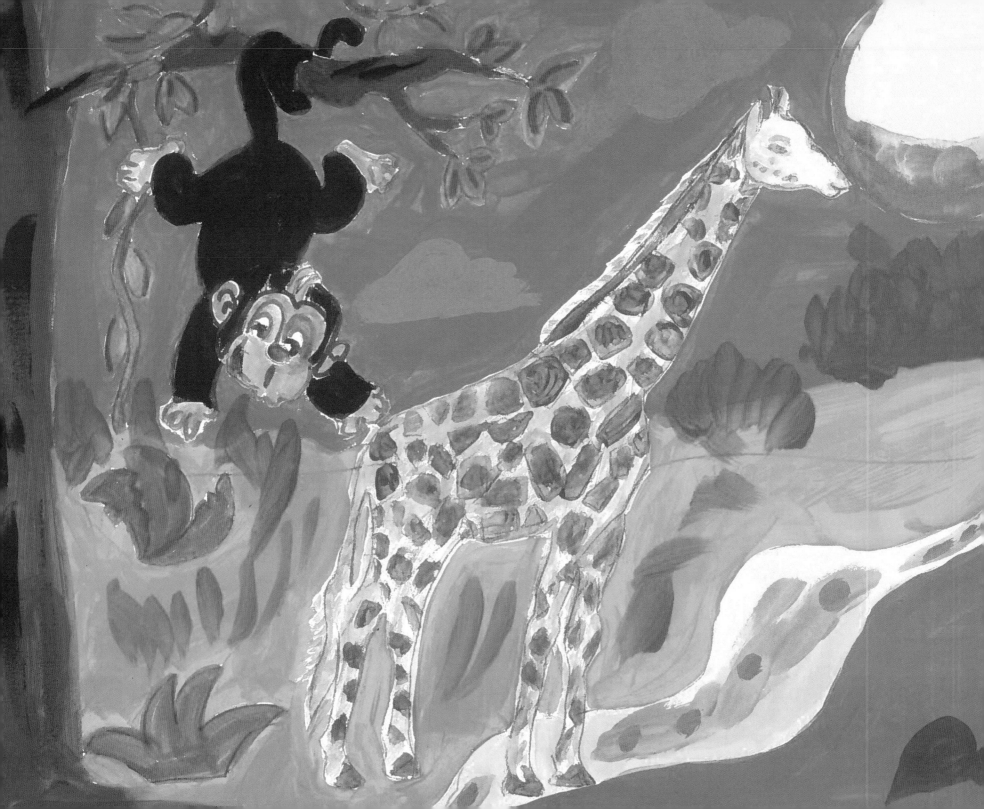

It wasn't long before Baby Duck could see his family with Sir Monkey hanging by his tail from a tree above them waiting for the little duck. It was quite the sight for Mama Duck to see her little baby on the back of a crocodile, even though Sir Monkey had told her about him being a vegan crocodile. All of the other ducklings were amazed at how impressive Baby Duck looked riding on top of a large croc.

"Mama, Mama!" proclaimed Baby Duck. He jumped off his vegan crocodile friend and swam into his mother's wings. After a good duck hug, he turned to Sir Monkey and said, "Thank you, Sir Monkey, for swinging ahead and letting my family know where we were."

"I am happy to be of service," bowed Sir Monkey still hanging from the tree by his tail.

As the duck family was reunited the sly tiger crouched down by the shore to better see the entire duck family. The tiger licked his lips while he watched the reunion with piercing eyes. 'This is my chance,' thought the sly tiger. 'Soon, I will be with a full stomach and have a duck feast all in one go.'

He crept up slowly so no-one would see of hear him. Just as everyone was saying their goodbyes, the sly tiger was becoming impatient. With a big tiger jump he leaped to the edge of the river bank and was just about to pounce on the Duck family.

Mama Duck saw the fierce Tiger and gathered her children, including Baby Duck, behind her. The vegan crocodile also saw the tiger and turned sharply to keep between the sly tiger and his new Duck friends.

The tiger tried to jump past the crocodile to snag the Duck family, but the vegan crocodile was too fast and could turn quickly in the water to keep the tiger at bay.

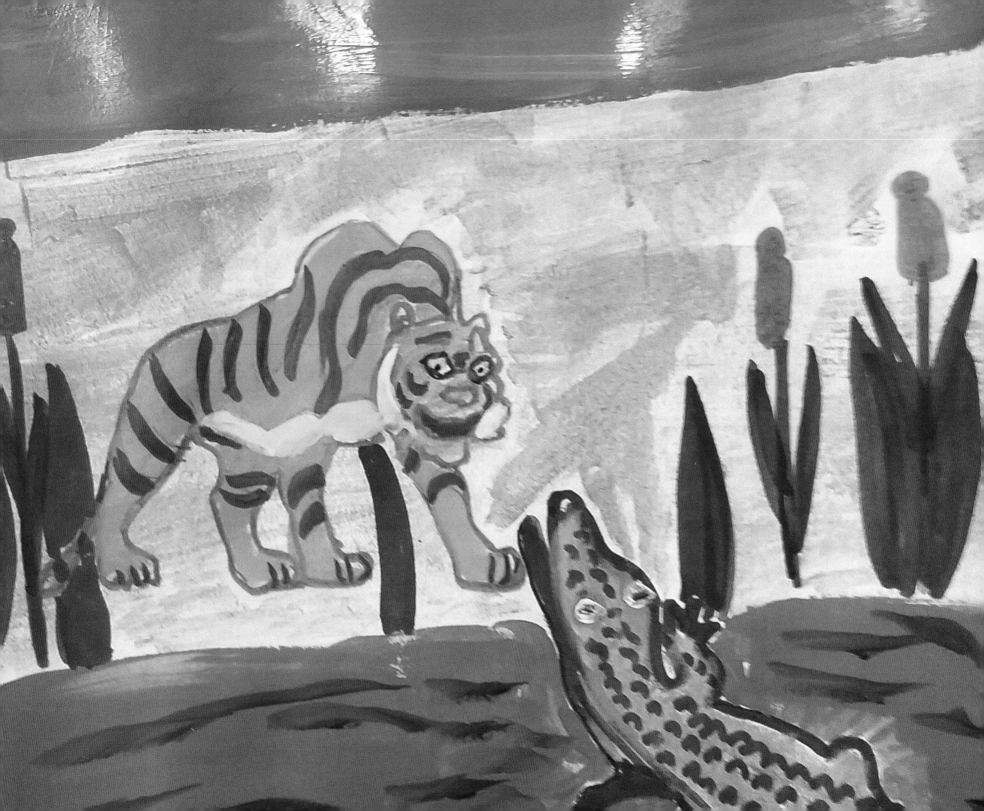

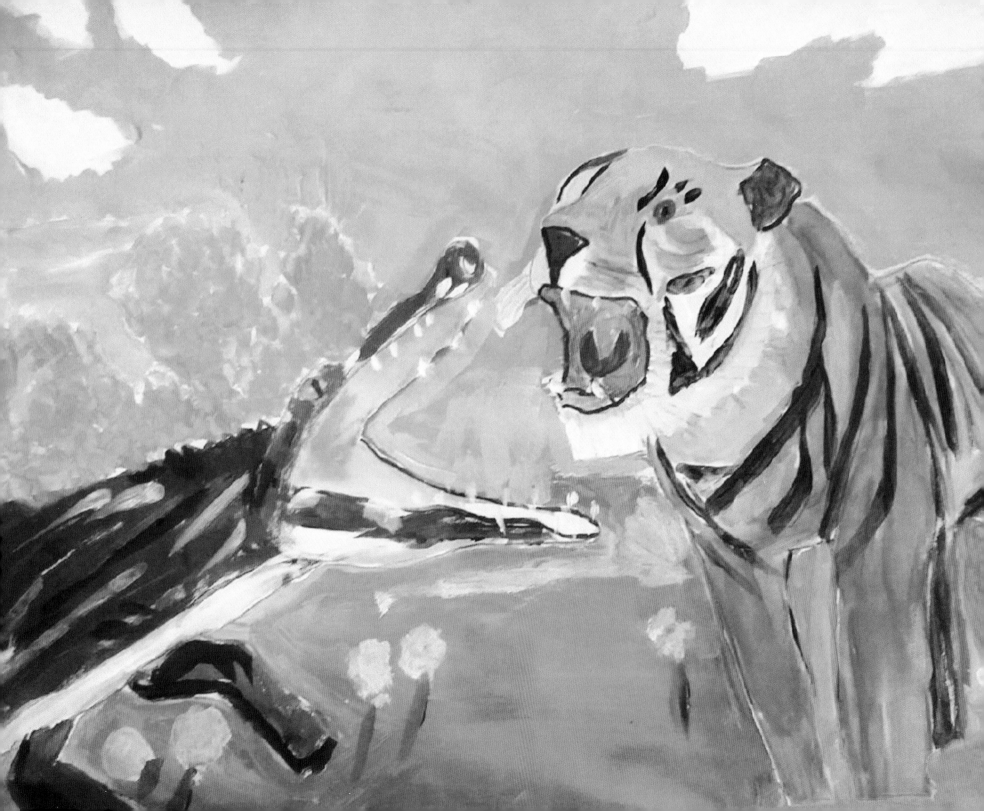

The frustrated sly tiger growled and roared but the vegan crocodile held his ground and hissed with his large mouth wide open showing his long sharp teeth.

Angry, the tiger yelled, "Don't you know that those ducks are food? Let me pass and I shall share them with you."

"Those ducks are my friends," braved the vegan crocodile. "They are not my food as I am a vegan and they aren't your food either! Now back off before I bite you on the nose." Enraged, the tiger gave up and ran off in the other direction, completely besides himself that a crocodile would save a family of ducks.

The duck family, Madam Giraffe, and Sir Monkey all celebrated the vegan crocodile's bravery. Baby Duck paddled over to his new friend. "The biggest thanks of all goes to you, Mr. Crocodile, for helping me find my family and saving all our lives." With that the Baby Duck gave the vegan crocodile a great big hug. A little crocodile tear could be seen sliding down the vegan crocodile's face.

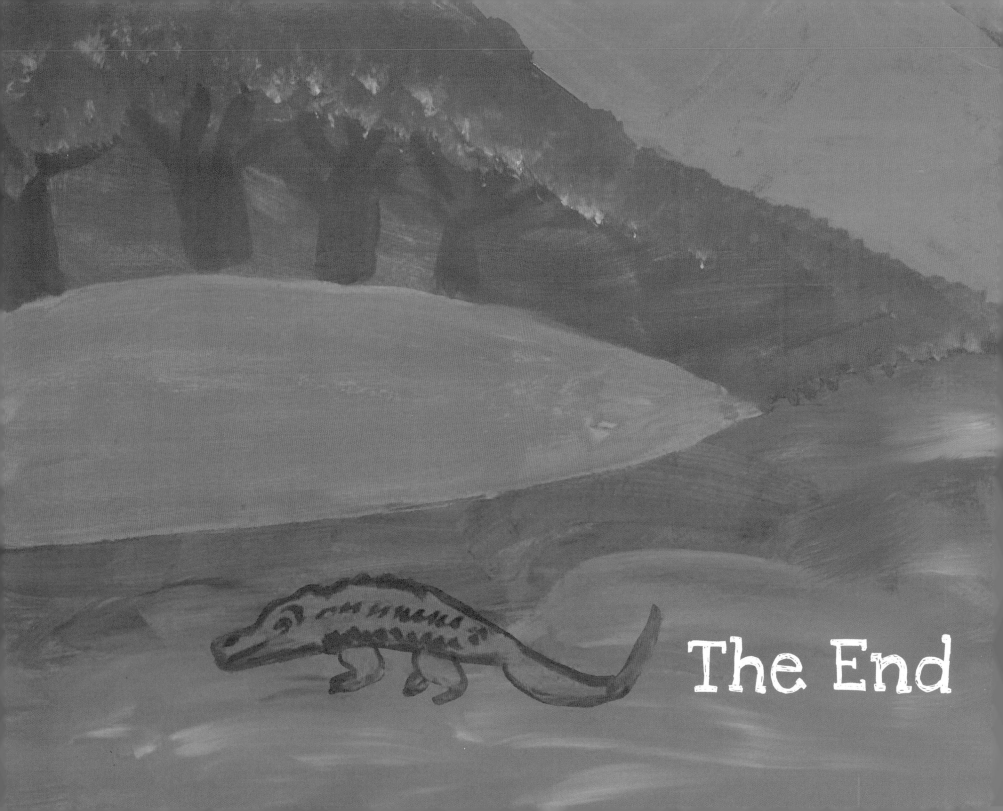

The End

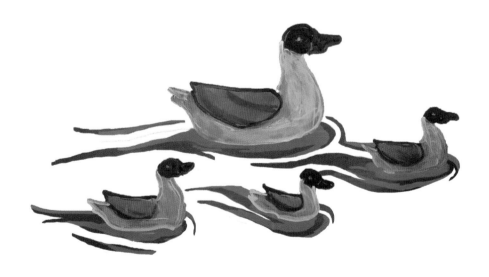

BRETT
LARK LLC

CPSIA information can be obtained at www.ICGtesting.com
Printed in the USA
LVIW011013140121
676460LV00005B/76